SENSATIONAL SLEEP

Better Sleep for a Better You

Stacey Duckett

SENSATIONAL SLEEP

Better Sleep for a Better You

Stacey Duckett

First Printing: May 2020

ISBN-13: 978-1-7370634-0-7

Beekeeper Publishing

A note to the Reader-Disclaimer:

This book is written and sold with the understanding that the author is not liable for any misconceptions. This book does not intend to be a substitute for consultation with a doctor or healthcare provider. The publisher and the author cannot claim any responsibility for any loss or damage caused or alleged, directly or indirectly, by the information contained in this book.

Table of Contents

FREE Sleep Assessment!

www.SensationalSleepBook.com

Would you like to get better sleep?

*FREE Sleep Assessment

*FREE Sleep Journal pdf

*Sign Up for FREE Email updates

*Join the group and share

Your SENSATIONAL SLEEP SUCCESS!

Stacey Duckett, D.C., A.C.N., CH, is available to speak at your business or conference event.

Visit: www.SensationalSleepBook.com

CHAPTER 1

No Sleep . . . Again

No sleep . . . again. Is that you? Are you busy and active all day long, but by the end of the day you are still wide awake? You lay down because you should be sleeping, but inside you cannot turn off the endless thoughts. You wish sound sleep were for you, but it seems you have lost the ability. You have been functioning with no sleep for quite some time, and you are just wondering when you are finally going to collapse. You even get nervous about driving in your car because you have not had much sleep. Difficulty with sleeping may start after having had a newborn and you never got back into the correct routine even once the kiddos went to school. For others, it could be a life-changing event such as death or divorce. Many women have difficulty sleeping due to menopause. For some endurance athletes, sleep problems happen once they take a sudden break from training. There are many reasons why one's sleep goes astray. Some may suffer from sleep apnea or a traumatic brain injury that needs follow-up with medical care such as a neurologist or a somnologist.

Have you reached the point where you are fed up enough with getting little sleep to do something about it? I am telling you that it would be foolish not to get your great sleep back in your life. Here is why. Without sleep, one is similar to a person driving under the influence. Many, if not all mental illnesses have one thing in common: sleep quality and quantity are not enough. If you lack sleep, you lose the ability to restore lessons. Your pain becomes constant. Your hormones that help with weight control do not work in your favor with the lack of sleep. You typically gain weight. Your blood pressure rises, and you are more likely to be diabetic as well. On top of this, your immune response suffers. The worst part of lack of sleep is that your cognitive function declines. Little sleep results in mood swings too. How well-functioning of a worker or employer, husband or wife, parent or child, student or teacher will you be? One can develop anxiety about going to sleep. You would think sleep is like drinking water. It should be a given something that comes naturally. Do you remember having consistent great nights of sleep? How long ago was it? How did you get so far off that it has come to this? You seriously need help to find a way to get your sleep, or you are going to go crazy! If this is you or someone you know, keep reading.

It happened to me. I was stressed and had some difficulty sleeping but nothing I could not handle—so I thought. It started after having kids. I'd stay up late or get up in the middle of the night, and then once my kids slept through, I would continue to get up in the middle of the night to do whatever. This habit went on for years. Then one day in my late 40s I was a bit stressed—single mom, self-employed—and I caught myself sitting in the chair realizing I hadn't taken a breath for a few minutes or more? And then realized, oh my gosh, I had to remind myself to breathe?! Silly thoughts but not so foolish when it is happening to you. What if this happens to me when I sleep? If I am sleeping and stop breathing, I won't be awake to remind myself to breathe. I felt disconnected with my automatic response for my body to function correctly—a misfire, like an automobile. The worry began. I started getting nervous about sleeping as if I maybe might not wake up. I would lay in bed, tossing and turning. I had completely given up caffeine at the time because of the issues with sleeping. In the past, if I did not have my cup of coffee in the morning, I would get a horrible headache. Something was different. I gave up the morning coffee, and I got no headache, and I was still wide awake. I felt like someone drugged me to stay awake, but no one had.

Worried that I would stop breathing during sleep, I went and got a sleep study. The test that I did was horrible. During the test I was required to wear a band around my head. The battery died, and I had a migraine for a week. I was curious about the results because it should show that I was dead since the battery died. Of course, I had no sleep

4

apnea. There are more accessible methods today to help determine if you have sleep apnea. Regardless, I was on a mission to solve this problem, or it would only be for a short while before I would collapse with an illness or some injury. The sleeping issue became so intense I started getting anxious about driving home from work, knowing it was only a short time before I would need to go to sleep. Has your insomnia gotten so bad where you, too, have strayed from having anxiety? The anxiety ended up with me choking at night almost every night for about three weeks. I thought I would die—if not in my sleep, then from choking. Before going to sleep, I would remind my girls where the life insurance papers were and tell them that I love them. Can you relate?

Through trial and error, I figured out what worked relatively quickly and then redefined and consistently improved my sleep. I came up with the acronym R.E.S.T. I will describe each acronym in further detail in this book. I can assure you that if you implement even one aspect of R.E.S.T., you too will get better sleep. REST—what does it stand for?

R for Routine

E for Ergonomics & posture-based exercise

S for Supplements with proper nutrition

T for Take out

Let's start with the ROUTINE that is a M.U.S.T.

M for Meditate

U for Under accountability

S for Strengths discovered and implemented into your daily life

T for Timely

I started this routine daily. The time I fall asleep might vary, but the time I wake up is the same. No naps. I made sure my routine was a M.U.S.T.:

Meditative state, prayer, self-hypnotic sleep session at night, or use an app like Calm.

Under accountability with a journal recording thoughts, dreams, and sleep habits.

Strength quiz was taken, and ways for implementation were found.

Timely sleep going to bed and waking up at the same time.

Ergonomics and exercise: I implemented correct ergonomics for the bedroom and day-to-day activities such as being at a desk and included specific exercises to improve posture.

Supplements and nutrition: with what boosted my overall health and promoted sleep.

Take out: I would take out of the picture what was not working in the bedroom or helping me fall asleep and stay asleep. Including myself, if I was not sleeping in 20 minutes.

R.E.S.T. helped me immensely to get a better quality and quantity of sleep. I became less stressed, had improved cognition, was not sore as often from exercising, and obtained better metabolism. Better sleep results in a better you. If you desire this for yourself, you will enjoy this book.

Why should you listen to me about sleeping better? It would be hard for me to take advice on running from a non-runner, but I could easily take the advice from someone who has trained to get into the Boston Marathon. Similarly, I would find it hard to take advice from one who has never struggled with sleep. I had issues with sleep and realized how it affects numerous aspects of our life. I have come up with steps to get you back on track via R.E.S.T.

As a Doctor of Chiropractic since 1992 and dealing with patients recovering from injuries, I realized that a lot of chronic pain was due to nutrition, exercise, thoughts, and sleep habits. Patients with proper sleep tend to recover quicker from injuries. If people continue with improper ergonomics in their day-to-day activities and the way they sleep, then less sleep and more pain prevail. Knowing that nutrition forms an integral part of how we feel and how we heal and sleep, I earned an Applied Clinical Nutritionist Certificate from Life Chiropractic West.

After having had my sleep issues, I furthered my studies and continue to do so on all aspects that would improve sleep. I became a Certified Hypnotist from the International Certification Board of Clinical Hypnotherapy, a Certified Sleep Science Coach from the Spencer Institute, and have completed a Certification in Sleep: Neurobiology, Medicine, and Society from the University of Michigan, Ann Arbor, Michigan. I also have a Certificate for Completion on The Science of Well-Being from Yale University—a series of challenges designed to increase your happiness and build more productive habits. With my education and discovering what works for better sleep, I have designed R.E.S.T.—Better Sleep for a Better You.

Read the following and ask yourself if you would like the same for yourself.

Mary was having a difficult time stopping all the continual thoughts at night. She was tossing and turning, she tried medications, but then the next day, she was out of it. R.E.S.T. helped her get her schedule back in sync. She is more alert, and the feeling of being overwhelmed has left her thoughts.

Candy, in her 50s, noticed she was approaching menopause. Candy started having more difficulty falling asleep and staying asleep. It wasn't enjoyable. She was gaining weight despite having worked out regularly and eating clean. R.E.S.T. helped her not just with sleep, but she noticed she started losing weight without changing her nutrition significantly to warrant an increased metabolism.

Kim, a professional businesswoman—a single Mom with two kids—was having difficulty with constant racing thoughts that she could not fall asleep for long before she would be up again. She tried many things and found using R.E.S.T. helped her to get better sleep. As a result, she can now stay calm and not get overworked. Her relationships with her kids and co-workers have improved immensely, and they have noticed a difference in her demeanor.

John, with his injury from years ago, started taking medications to help him sleep. The meds began to stop working. He would try others, and they were way too strong where he was then not functioning the next day, or they did not work. His sleep got worse. Fortunately, he found R.E.S.T. to be beneficial. Through the program, he was referred to other professionals as well, like the dentist. He was happy to receive the recommendation, and with the accountability, it helped make sure he was on top of his commitment to improving his sleep. He now falls asleep shortly after lying in bed, and he stays asleep for the entire night.

Fay stopped drinking caffeinated drinks, stopped her sugar intake, and she still had insomnia. Fay wanted to avoid taking medications as far as possible. Because Fay was not getting quality sleep, she frequently noticed to be getting sleepy while driving. It got so bad she would have to pull off the road to take a mini-nap when she heard about R.E.S.T. from a friend—and decided to not only get her sleep but also her life back. That was the best decision ever. Her sleep has improved. She can stay awake during the day and not be worried about falling asleep, especially while driving.

You, too, can achieve great sleep—both quality and quantity. I guarantee that if you implement R.E.S.T., your life will be better. Turn to the next chapter and continue to read and implement this into your own life so you can achieve a night of better sleep for a better you.

CHAPTER 2

Why Are You Having Difficulty Sleeping?

D o you remember a time in which you were able to lay down and quickly fall asleep? What happened? How did you lose the ability to sleep? Sleep should naturally occur. Well, the answer is yes, provided your sleep-wake circadian rhythm is functioning. Circadian rhythm is a 24-hour clock running in your background. This cycle works via light signals through your eyes, with the sunlight telling you to be awake and via darkness telling your system to go to sleep. If it goes astray, insomnia can occur. Your circadian rhythm ensures your body will function properly at the right time. All circadian rhythms connect to your master clock, the Supra

Chiasmatic Nucleus (S.C.N.), which is part of the brain's hypothalamus. The sleep-wake cycle can be affected by several different elements such as exercise, activities, stress, room temperature, and travel to a different time zone. The one element that influences the S.C.N. most significantly is light. There are various reasons why insomnia can occur. Most of you are having trouble falling asleep because there is just too much light at night. If you change this one aspect alone, your sleep will improve. We are on our phones, computers, and TVs to the wee hours of the night. Want to reset your sleep? Try going camping in the tent in the fall with colder weather to a place where there is no extra light or Wi-Fi. You will naturally be tired quicker than if you were at home—simply because there isn't the light. For some, you lost your routine: a new mom or a graveyard shift worker. Perhaps you suffered from a traumatic brain injury (T.B.I.) from a motor vehicle collision, a fall, or a sports-related injury. These injuries may affect the S.C.N. that then leads to not allowing one to perceive light signals correctly. Melatonin production decreases, resulting in less sleep and increased fatigue with a traumatic brain injury. A recent death in the family or a divorce or suffering from Post-Traumatic Stress Disorder can make it difficult to sleep. P.T.S.D. increases epinephrine and adrenaline in the brain, leading to frequent naps during the day, making sleeping at night even more problematic.

Poor posture can create havoc on your sleep via a negative feedback loop. If one has a forward head posture that most do, then contracture occurs in the neck muscles. Your posture can lead to you breathing more through your mouth than your nose. Breathing through your mouth can lead to sleep apnea. We have more oxygen to the brain with nose breathing. With mouth breathing, there is less oxygen to your brain which results in less restful sleep. Later, we will discuss correcting your body's faulty biomechanics, workstation, and bedroom to enhance your sleep. We will discuss specific stretches that help reduce forward head posture.

Being overworked and stressed causes your cortisone hormone to increase, keeping you wired at night and melatonin declines, worsening your ability to fall asleep and stay asleep.

Electromagnetic frequencies, EMFs—research suggests they affect your sleep by reducing your melatonin. If you wear a "smartwatch" to know your sleep cycle, maybe use it for a week, then consider turning it off. Why take the risk, turn off the Wi-Fi, the blue tooth, the cellular. Your alarm will still work, but better yet, you could use a wind-up watch with an alarm instead. There is a demand for more studies on this topic. If you are on social medial, shopping online, or watching the news, and the stress of all that is going on with bombardment of thoughts, it would be much better to do a crossword puzzle or read a book. Give yourself time to take a break.

Maybe you are going through menopause.⬜ Low estrogen levels reduce the ability of magnesium to get into tissues. A reduction of magnesium in the tissues reduces getting the sleep neurotransmitters such as melatonin to function. You will have a hard time falling asleep and staying asleep. The fluctuating hormones may also cause hot flashes that can wake up the brain at night, causing one difficulty to get more R.E.M. sleep.

Athletes that suddenly stop training often can get insomnia. Like being overworked and stressed, an endurance athlete can have cortisol increase and remain high with high levels of training and weeks leading up to the race and even after the race.

Traveling to different time zones—similar to graveyard shift workers—can cause sleep disruption. When traveling, our circadian rhythms often stay on their original biological schedule for several days if at a new time zone.

For many, it may simply be from just not getting enough sun during the day. Not enough sunlight will decrease your cortisol during the day and then too much light at night causes your cortisol to increase, inhibiting melatonin from being produced when it is dark.

For others, it is too much caffeine. Caffeine can have a disruptive effect on your sleep. The stimulant's most apparent effect is that it can make it hard for you to fall asleep. One study also found that caffeine can delay the timing of your body clock. These effects will reduce your total sleep time. Caffeine also can reduce the amount of deep sleep that you enjoy.

The effects of caffeine can occur even when you consume it earlier in the afternoon or evening. One study found that consuming caffeine 6 hours before bedtime reduced total sleep time by 1 hour.

People tend to be more tense and have difficulty sleeping if they are stressed or depressed. Studies show that in improving your mood, one should not focus solely on the pathology but to discover your strengths and then use them. People who suffer from this tend not to be implementing their strengths into their life. Once you find out your talents, you may not even realize what is unique about you and when using them people tend to feel better. Even if you are not in a job you love it is still essential to know your strengths and find a way to use them daily to give you some peace. With peace, one will find it easier to sleep. Studies show that sleep affects mood, and mood affects sleep. Although sleep tends to affect mood greater than the other, it is crucial to assess your mood and improve it.

Some people suffer from various problems such as sleep apnea, causing one to stop breathing while sleeping, interfering with R.E.M. sleep. People tend to be overweight because they are not getting enough R.E.M. sleep. Their hormones for Ghrelin and Leptin are out of sync. The excess weight makes it more difficult to breathe, and the cycle continues. Sleep centers can have you take a sleep test in-house or take-home equipment or try apps to determine if this is what you have. Some people have alignment issues with their gums or Tori overgrown gum, making the tongue not have room to rest in the bottom of the mouth. Seeking out a dentist for mouth guards or oral surgeons may also prove to be helpful.

Many reasons people get insomnia, including poor diet, leads to one having an increase in inflammation. An increase in inflammation tends to one getting poor quality of sleep.

Currently, one in two thousand Americans suffers from narcolepsy. These people suddenly fall asleep at the wrong time. Some have cataplexy, where the muscles stop functioning, and they collapse. These conditions need to be under medical care.

When researching animals, it looks like domestic animals also can get insomnia. Mammals in the wild often do not get insomnia unless fearing for life—then they can. Some birds can sleep with one eye open, resting half of their brain while the other half remains alert. It's called unihemispheric slow-wave sleep. Some mammals like dolphins have one half brain sleeping while the other is awake to go up to the surface to breathe. Humans can get this as a first-night effect of sleeping in a different place.

Most people with insomnia have more than one factor causing the issue. I challenge you to change one thing and notice how it can improve your sleep.

Insomniacs may not necessarily be interested in the why and how sleep occurs. They want to be able to fall asleep and stay asleep. They want results. However, it may help to focus on why it is so essential to improving your sleep, hence motivating you to push forward to enhance your sleep with a basic understanding.

There is a lot of literature on sleep, yet we still need to learn more about it. In this book, I reference some scientific studies.⬚ This book is not to inundate you with scientific research but a simple way to remember steps on improving your sleep.⊠ If you are interested in a more detailed analysis, I suggest the book Why We Sleep.⊠ Studies mentioned in the book Why We Sleep demonstrate why quality and quantity of sleep matter.

If the circadian rhythm is functioning correctly, you will get quality and quantity of sleep. With the correct functioning circadian rhythm, you will have a night of better sleep, resulting in better immunity, metabolism, focus, and mobility. Getting enough proper light during the day increases serotonin allowing one to be wakeful and getting signals that the day is over via darkness increases melatonin to allow for sleep.

The bottom line is that these various reasons resulting in a lack of sleep cause a⊠decline in one or more of your hormones that either hinders sleep or promotes⊠alertness.⊠⊠

What makes this book different is that it puts it all together using an easy-to-remember acronym, R.E.S.T.—addressing the issues behind why we have difficulty sleeping and how to change for the better. If you start with the R and work on that alone, I promise you will improve your sleep.

CHAPTER 3

What Happens with Lack of Sleep?

No sleep affects you harmfully. Sensational sleep affects you significantly. Before we get into what happens with lack of sleep, let's briefly discuss sleep phases. Each step is vital in getting sensational sleep.

There are 4 phases of sleep, and they are:

Stage 1: Sleep is light and easy to wake from.

Stage 2: Brain waves start to slow down.

Stages 3 & 4: Deeper sleep. It will be more challenging to wake up during this time. Restorative sleep.

Rapid eye movement (R.E.M.): During the final stage in the sleep cycle, your brain becomes more active, and dreams occur. Your brain is processing information and storing long-term memories.

This cycle repeats every 90 to 110 minutes. R.E.M. cycles increase in length as sleep continues.

When there is a lack of sleep with quality, quantity, or both, several harmful activities can occur.

Blood pressure increases with lack of sleep. Sleep helps allow your body to balance hormones. If your hormones dealing with stress are not normalized, your blood pressure may rise, and if your metabolism slowed down and you gain weight, it will also lead to your blood pressure increasing.

Hormones out of whack. Lack of sleep increases the hormone Ghrelin, so you feel hungry. It decreases the Leptin hormone, which makes one feel full. Hence lack of sleep, one gains weight. If you get better quality and quantity of sleep, your metabolism can increase, shedding unwanted pounds. People with sleep apnea have a lack of adequate sleep and are overweight. The increase in weight increases the problem with breathing, and the increase in mouth breathing can result in sleep apnea.

Numerous studies demonstrate that the less you sleep, the less you can remember. Diminished sleep even after one night causes an increase in beta-amyloid in the brain.

Beta-amyloid forms by the breakdown of larger protein molecules that in a healthy brain would be removed from the brain, but with lack of sleep, the brain does not remove them. They stick together and create havoc. Beta-amyloid you will find in Alzheimer's disease. When one is not getting adequate sleep, there is inhibition in mitochondrial metabolism and decreased neuron membranes' excitability in the brain. Without these neuron membranes turning on sufficiently then there is a difficulty remembering.

Diabetes rises with lack of sleep. When one gets less sleep, the blood sugar increases, a precursor to diabetes; you can read this in the book Why We Sleep by Dr. Walker.

Lack of sleep results in moodiness and mental problems such as anxiety and depression. Lack of sleep studies shows an increased moodiness. When sleep restores, the sense of well-being improves significantly.

Lack of sleep results in decreased immunity. Scientific studies show that people with less quality and or quantity of sleep are more likely to catch a virus like a cold and that it will also be more challenging and take longer for you to recover. T cells have less ability to fight, and fewer cytokines are released to help you fight infection.

Lack of sleep results in increased pain and decreased inability to repair and restore from injuries. Sleep deprivation impairs functional muscle recovery following an injury.

With adequate sleep, growth hormone releases during deep sleep.⬜ Helping with helping and repair if you are not getting deep sleep, then how will you heal?⬜ One enters R.E.M. typically every 90 minutes of sleep.⬜ Hence the quantity of how long you sleep is essential. You will have more opportunities to enter R.E.M.⬜ R.E.M. allows one to acknowledge what has occurred during the day and situations that need handling to process deep strategic solving insights.⯑⯑

Lack of sleep decreases your life expectancy because you tend to gain weight, increases blood glucose with a higher risk of diabetes, and tend to higher amounts of inflammation, causing cardiovascular disease, resulting in decreased life expectancy. If you lack sleep, imperatively you will want to improve on this aspect of your life. An increase in inflammatory responses has increased with lack of quality and quantity of sleep—in experiments and associations noted with many diseases. Therefore, achieving sensational sleep is prudent to your well-being.

Screening tools to find sleep disturbances and setting up excellent sleep hygiene is imperative to our society. Reducing systemic inflammation by the food we eat and supplements we take can be helpful.

If you lack sleep or sleep quality, it is good to know where you are specifically having issues. Maybe you think you have a significant quantity of sleep but are still tired, not ready to start the day. It would be good to consider investing in an Oura

Sleep Tracking Ring, or some may have an Apple Watch with a sleep tracking device. Some reading this book may want better quantity sleep. These devices can help you clue where you are lacking and help set you up for a routine. For some, wearing a device while you sleep makes you conscious and worried about it working or has enough charge or being too loose. One is left wondering will the reading be accurate. Or if you get up in the middle of the night, you catch yourself checking to see if the device picked up on that or not. The thoughts start getting in the way of you just sleeping. Wearing a device can give you information about where you are and where you would like to be. Keep in mind that a sleep tracker can assume how much R.E.M. and Non-R.E.M. sleep you got. The only way to accurately identify what stage of sleep you are in is during a clinical sleep study measuring your brain activity with a polysomnography. Currently, the consumer devices do not count this activity precisely. They make an assumption based on your lack of movement, the rate of your heart and respiration rate, and rhythm that you must be in a particular phase of sleep. During non-R.E.M. sleep, your heart rate, breathing, and blood pressure drop to levels below those while you are awake. R.E.M. is the stage of sleep when your blood pressure and heart rate can go up and down during this stage. They base this on that heart rate and respiration rates have a close relationship with each sleep stage. For instance, in a deep sleep, your respiration rate is shallow and varied.

The algorithm used in measuring sleep stages based on cardiac function may differ based on age, sex, and even the location of where you are.

Some people may look at their wearable device data and think they are getting great sleep but genuinely are not. I think though we all know if we are getting enough sleep or not. By asking questions such as do I wake up refreshed? Can I remember things, or do I have brain fog? Am I overweight? Is my body able to recover from sickness or an injury, or is it taking seemingly longer than it should be? Is my blood pressure high? If you answered yes to any of these or no, or is someone who can say yes to one of these questions, you might want to get an Oura Sleep Tracking Ring or sleep app. I have both the watch and the ring. For me, I like the ring because it is nonintrusive. However, the watch keeps me on track for bedtime alarms and use when training for a running race.

Some of you who have sleep apnea could go into sleep study where they wire you up.

Sleep devices have lights on them that may keep you up, and studies hopefully in the future will help determine if having this technology on all the time is safe for you to wear day in and night out. However, wearing the device might help you get your sleep back into a routine and clue you in why you are not getting great sleep. I also believe in the old-fashioned way of writing it down and seeing it for myself in a journal. We will talk about that in the next chapter.

Now that we have discussed how you lost the ability to sleep and what happens with not enough sleep continue to read to implementing R.E.S.T.— an acronym for you to get better sleep for a better you.

You are improving your R.E.S.T. to enhance your sleep resulting in improved cognition, metabolism, immunity, mood, life expectancy, and even mobility.

R is for Routine that is a M.U.S.T.

E is for Ergonomics and Exercise

S is for Supplements

T is for Taking out what does not work for you

Next chapter, we will start with your Routine, and including the M.U.S.T. will have a significant impact on your sleep and, therefore, your life.

CHAPTER 4

How Do You Get Your Sleep Back?

How do you get your sleep back? Start with your ROUTINE.

What should my guidelines be for my routine? A great therapist will recommend the top item to do is to set up a practice. A therapist may use Cognitive Behavior Therapy and Eye Movement Desensitization Re-education Therapy to help sleep.

Digital Cognitive Behavioral Therapy study reported in Jama shows that it can help significantly with insomnia.

The number one thing one can do is to start a routine and stick to it. You stick to it regardless of if it is a weekend or a holiday. Your health is too crucial to mess with it.

Three exceptions to NO NAPS.

One: if you are a new Mom, maybe two years of napping for this group is okay. Get your sleep the best you can, however you can.

Two: graveyard shift folks, the best you can, again stick to the routine, whether working or not. Best for you to fool yourself into thinking day is night, and night is day. Literally, regarding your health, I doubt if you are getting paid enough. Working during the typical hours one should be sleeping takes a toll on your mental and physical health. For graveyard shift workers, if you are not falling asleep or staying asleep throughout the night, I would take naps.

Three: death, major illness, or significant stress trigger for a short period of 1–2 weeks; get a nap where you can.

For everyone else, set up a routine, so you innately know when to sleep and naturally awake. Sleeping during the hours from 10:00 p.m. to 2:00 a.m. is a bonus because of restorative sleep time. Restorative time is when melatonin and growth hormone are high and helps clean your body, remove debris, and restore it. During the day, Adenosine builds up. By the end of the day, it helps to tell you that you are tired and need to sleep. Amyloid beta is also created in the brain and needs sleep to clean this debris out.

Your routine should be **M.U.S.T.**

M - Meditative. Part of your routine should be meditative. A simple mantra, a prayer said over and over. You could use a meditative app. or a hypnotic recording. Perhaps even one you recorded yourself. It's something powerful to hear in your voice a guided hypnotic state. Record your thoughts from the day by writing down issues that you would like to resolve in a journal before you sleep at night. When you combine this with stating I will get sensational sleep tonight and I will wake up with solutions to improve in the areas I wrote upon can be powerful. Meditation helps to reduce cortisol and increase melatonin. Studies have shown in older adults comparing meditation alone versus set routine not including meditation—those receiving mediation slept better in older adults. That is why I believe your routine needs to include a form of meditation. A meditation could consist of a self-hypnosis technique. Hypnosis . . . do not let it scare you; hypnosis in Greek means sleep. By reading the script below, we want you to see there is nothing scary about it. For example, here is one that I like to implement that I am sharing with you with slight changes with permission from Dr. Richard Nongard. I have taped it and listened to it at night on particular nights that I found it difficult to sleep—it is a way to start the sleep cycle going by getting yourself to a trance-like state. Hearing in your voice is helping you take command of your mind.

In hypnosis, we first start with progressive muscle relaxation. Record yourself and fill in your name:

_____. You are going to be guided through a relaxation state. All you need to do at this moment is to make yourself very comfortable, and you can move as you need to as you proceed to get in even a further state of comfort. _____ simply just close your eyes. Take inventory where you may have any tension in your body and commit yourself to release that tension. You want all the muscles in your body to relax. As you relax, notice that your breath has already started to become slower. This is good. Take a deep breath in for 4, and release for 6 counts. Deep, slow breaths help us to get into a state of relaxation and hypnosis. Very good. As you relax more fully and get even more comfortable, imagine letting go of the tension in the muscles in the top of your head, your brow, muscles around your eyes and jaw, and even the muscles around your mouth. Release the tension in the muscles of your face and the top of your head.

_____as you allow your body to experience a state of physical relaxation, do not worry if your mind wanders. Just come back, focus on your deep breaths in for 4, and let go for 6. Continue to release the tension in your body along your shoulders, arms, and upper back. You will likely feel the tension come down from your upper back down your arms to your hands and out of your fingertips. Any stress of the day: visualize it leaving your body. Focus on the muscles in your chest, stomach, and your lower back. If any of these muscles are tense, simply let go of it. Your muscles are becoming loose and limp, like a big pile of rubber bands. You experience sensational relaxation. This brings you even to a deeper state. Relaxing the mind is now an easy thing to do. As your body relaxes, your mind becomes more relaxed.

Your legs do a lot of work for you. The tension of the day can store up in the muscles along the hip, buttocks, or your upper leg. Let this tension simply flow from your thighs and calves, the muscle of the feet, ankles and out of your toes. At this time _____ you are very relaxed. If you need to swallow or adjust for comfort, that's okay. Congratulations _____ from your head to your toes, you have allowed yourself to become completely relaxed.

Your mind is also able to completely relax, just like your body. This skill allowing your mind to relax will help you to apply to many areas of your life to help come up with solutions to issues you may be struggling with. With your current feeling of deep relaxation perhaps you could feel like you could open your eyes if you wanted but this feels so good you simply continue to choose to keep them closed. Enjoy this blissful feeling for a moment. (Pause)

As you allow your body to become limp, loose and relaxed, this will become meaningful to you. Meaningful because you _____ have acquired a new skill: the skill of taking control over your own body and mind. (Pause)

Sleep Script

Although you are not asleep, you can use this state of hypnosis to shift from external distractions to a point of calmness. The mind is quite powerful. You may be aware of many experiences at this point, including the room temperature, sounds from outside, and others nearby. In the past, these noises may have distracted you, but now you can recognize that you have the ability to shift your awareness to any experience, including those you create in your mind. The mind has a place deep inside of it where awareness is created. Until hearing this, perhaps you were unaware of this place. However, now that you know about it, you can shift your awareness from all that is outside of you to this place in the mind.

From here you can use the creative part of your mind to begin to drift, dream and float inside of your own awareness. You can use the creative part of the mind to envision yourself, perhaps under a clear blue sky. Perhaps you are in a beautiful place you have been to before, a place that you would like to go or even a place you have created that is relaxing and peaceful. Wonderful!

Imagine that as you look to the clear blue sky, you can see a single white puffy cloud gently floating by. See the soft edges of the cloud and the pure energy of its radiance. Watch as it gently moves from one side of the sky to the other. Imagine that all of your stress, discomfort, or concerns become enveloped by the energy in this cloud.

As the cloud moves into the horizon, becomes smaller and smaller, you become increasingly aware of your mind's ability to relax and create its own experiences. It has long forgotten about any difficulties that used to concern you. It will eventually become so small that it completely disappears. At this point, you are sensing an awareness of your feelings of deepening relaxation. Do you feel yourself moving twice as deep into relaxation of mind and body? Go all the way down into deep mental relaxation. Perfect. With a sense of security and comfort, you could be happy about the new experience as a lesson you have had that can help you to sleep deeply at night.

I'm going to give you some suggestions now you can pay attention to each and every word with your conscious mind or you can drift, dream, and float. You can hear all the words of the subconscious mind and only every other word, every fifth word, or every tenth word with the conscious mind. Perfect. These are suggestions that you have asked me to make when you asked me to help you sleep better, so they are suggestions that come from you. You will find it easy to internalize an experience the suggestions now and anytime you need a restful night of deep tranquility. Each night as you experience self-hypnosis, you will find it easier to follow the instructions and you're more deeply into trance and eventually into sleep.

As you listen to your breathing and perhaps think about the sweet, soft sounds of nature, you begin to move your thoughts from those that are external to those that are inside the part of the mind where creativity and awareness are created. This will allow you to detach from anything that previously harmed your sleep.

As you continue to relax, let yourself freely and lazily double the sensation of relaxation in both mind and body, let go of any tension in any muscle. This feeling of the loosening of the muscles will bring you even further into a trance. You know that at this moment you could open your eyes or wake up entirely, but it feels so good to finally let go that you will continue to do exactly what you're now doing and experience an even deeper level of hypnosis or relaxation. Although you know you have the ability to awaken if something needs to be attended to, at this point, there are no outside concerns. Therefore, it is okay to let yourself go deeper and deeper into trance.

In the morning when it's time to wake yourself, your journal winners of the freshness of a new day will bring an energy and sense of wellness that will carry you through tomorrow. It's wonderful to feel refreshed and revived from a good night of sleep, however, this time does not now end. It is perfectly okay to continue focusing your awareness inward and eventually drifting from hypnosis into deep sleep. Count backwards from 10 to 1, enjoy the feeling of heaviness in the arms and legs, the feeling of coolest of all the desire and the sensation of rest in both mind and body—ten rest, nine perfect, eight peace, seven slowly drifting into sleep—nine, eight, seven, six, with each number not knowing where sleep begins . . . Seven . . . Six, just experiencing the process . . . Five, good . . . Four . . . Three, total comfort . . . Four, safe . . . three . . . Two, wonderful . . . One, drifting to a point where awareness of awareness simply drifts off into the distance . . . Sleep . . .

I hope you make a self-prerecorded self-hypnosis such as this one and start using it tonight.

U **- Under Accountability.** Use a sleep tracking device mentioned in the previous chapter like the Oura Ring, a sleep coach, or, if it works for you, a journal specifically for sleep. I recommend writing your thoughts for the day and any issues you'd like to resolve. Your meditation or hypnosis could encourage a mantra such as "I will have a restful and restorative sleep. Any problems I have, I will receive some solutions tonight." You may remember them when you awake and can record your progress and use the wisdom you have discovered to decide how to proceed with the day. Dreams are keys, and we have gotten away from this. If the third of our time we spend on sleep, it is good to reflect on those dreams that were so vivid. Writing down those thoughts when you wake up will start to impress on you to remember. Solutions can come from yourself if you open yourself up to your subconscious mind. While obtaining my sleep coach certificate through the Spencer Institute, there was an interview with author Justina Lasley—the Institute for Dream Studies founder. Her book Wake up to Your Dreams Transform Your Relationships, Career, and Health While You Sleep is a fantastic read with great insight.

S - Strengths. Part of one not sleeping well may be that you are not utilizing your strengths daily. If you are not using your strengths, you are stifling.

Stifling leads to stress. If you are unsure of your strengths, take this quiz at www.viacharacter.org; after you complete the questions, it will populate the list of your top strengths. Finding a way to utilize your top 3 in your day-to-day activities, including your work, will help you feel more in tune with fewer frustrations. Feeling that you live your life optimally using your given talents helps one reduce racing thoughts at night that keep you awake. Research has shown that using your strengths allows one to sleep better to get sensational sleep.

T - Timely. You must start your bedtime routine every night at the same time and wake up in the morning at the same time. You must be sleeping within 20 minutes. If you are not, get out of the bedroom and do something relaxing. Maybe crossword puzzles or reading books or writing. Keep in mind this is not for you to do in your bedroom. You need to quickly get your brain to realize that your bed is not where you have racing thoughts, toss and turn, or watching TV. Your bedroom is for sleeping and having sex. If you are not doing either of those, then leave the room until you feel sleepy again. The catch is that you still need to get up in the morning as scheduled. There are NO NAPS unless you are sick, mom with little ones or have had a brain injury. This way, that day and maybe the next couple of days or weeks will be difficult, but soon enough, your brain will begin to be the program that you are sleeping or having sex when you hit the sack. Maybe best to have sex then sleep because sex helps one sleep.

Summarizing R for routine in R.E.S.T. with acronym M.U.S.T.

M - Meditative

U - Under Accountability

S - Strengths

T - Timely

CHAPTER 5

Ergonomics and Exercise, Your Ergonomics

Ergonomics of your day can be the cause of your aches and pains. People who are in pain have a more difficult time falling asleep and staying asleep. People who sleep less tend not to recover from their injuries because they do not get restorative sleep. Poor ergonomics during the day and at night for many leads one to forward head posture. People often commute with not their heads resting on the headrest but leaning forward. Many people work at a desk with their heads bent forward. Others work with their head down like a chiropractor or a dentist. Students often study with their heads bent forward. Many people, not just students and teens, have developed text necks.

Another name for forward head posture. Many people consistently overuse their shoulder and upper extremity, usually their dominant side. One with forward head posture is more likely to have the neck muscles contract, muscles in the front constrict, and the muscles in the back of the neck to overstretch. I often have a patient hold an actual bowling ball close to their chest and then have them hold it with their arms extended. Even imagining this one can acknowledge how it is so much easier if the weight is closer to you than further away from the body. Same as your head on your spine. If your head is too far forward, the back of the neck muscles will strain. The neck muscle in front needs to stretch. The neck muscles in the back could benefit significantly from myofascial release and chiropractic adjustments of the cervical spine. This work helps correct the spine's faulty biomechanics. The following muscles constrict with forward head posture: the Scalenes, Sternocleidomastoid, Pectoralis Major, and the Pectoralis Minor. The muscle in the back of the neck and upper back that tend to overstretch is the Trapezius and Levator Scapulae.

Breathing better can help improve your core muscles, helping guard your lower back to help reduce low back pain and help you sleep better. A forward head posture leads one to breathe more from the chest than deep breathing. Ultimately one will tend to breathe through the mouth instead of the nose. The Scalene muscles help to elevate the ribs. The Scalene muscles attach from the vertebrae in the cervical spine to the first and second rib. The function of this muscle is to help elevate the ribs. With the muscle unable to work correctly, it leads to one breathing more through their mouth. Forward head posture also tends to lead one to gain weight and snoring, putting further pressure on your ability to breathe in fully. Correcting your ergonomics during the day will help; however, it can be beneficial to seek out chiropractic care to help your joints move correctly especially if you have been chronically out of alignment. Technology has come a long way. It can look at your posture statically and through motion; you sit at your desk to how you walk and move. In my own office, we use the app Posture Screen. Many chiropractors and Physical Therapists use this in their office. It is a great tool to have for yourself. You see for yourself on a grid your posture. You can see how forward your head is from the rest of the spine. You can view if you are leaning to left or right or rotating in your neck or back. When people see how their posture truly is, they can assess what might be causing this to occur and make changes during the day. It may not just be what they are doing during the day but also how they are sleeping at night contributing to this forward head posture and other postural deviations. After having a full day of forward head posture activities, some people go home to go to sleep eventually and then use an overstuffed pillow that causes their head to remain in a forward head posture. Some people sleep on their sides but have their head tilt prop up too high or too low. It should be 90 degrees. The middle of your ear should be over the middle of the spine. So, your neck is even with the rest of the spine. Stomach sleeping is the worst for your neck. Stomach sleepers often will sleep night after night, week after week, month after month, year after year with their head turned to the same side. Have you ever been to a concert, and you had to sit at an angle only to find your neck hurting the next day? If you are a stomach sleeper, try turning your head both ways and lay down. Does one side feel stuck like it is not as flexible? Often this is due to muscles stretched on one side and constricted on the other side. Tools like the Posture Screen App can help you see the problems you are having with your ergonomics. Once you optimize your ergonomics, you can again reassess and continue to do this until your posture balances to the best of its capability, given each one's consideration of the activity they engage in day in and day out.

As a chiropractor, I often get asked which pillow is the best for me? I have gone through various pillows to sell to customers. The answer is the one you sleep best on and helps you maintain proper posture allowing you to breathe easier and recover from the stress put on your body, especially your neck, throughout the day. One pillow that I have taken a liking to is the Coop Pillow. It is CertiPUR-US and GREENGUARD Gold. It allows you to remove foam inside or add foam to get a great fit so that your posture is correct. It is helpful to have someone assess this as you lay on the pillow, or you could use a mirror or set up an automatic photo. Some people get a cold or have difficulty sleeping flat and like to prop up their heads higher than their chest. In this case, try using the wedge pillow or another pillow as the base and then take a rolled-up towel placed under your neck so you maintain the ear's opening to be aligned with the middle of the shoulder when sleeping on your back.

Sleeping on a great mattress is again one that you sleep well on and that when you wake up, you should feel great. You should feel restored. Unfortunately, people do get degenerative arthritis, and they will often wake up in pain, and then as the day goes on, as their body warms up, the pain lessens. Having a great bed that discovers where it can automatically adjust the firmness to get the best sleep is a fantastic idea. Several mattress companies are out there that will allow you to try it and see if it is a good fit for you or not for so many days. Some days, you worked out hard, and maybe a softer bed would be appealing to the typical day where you would be better off with a firmer mattress. I like the idea of having your sleep monitored to help recommend what the best is but with having you also be able to change to suit your needs at the time. There are Tempurpedic beds, but often, people have a difficult time getting off from them. There are air beds and hybrid beds. One that gets a lot of recognition is the Sleep Number 360 Bed.

Ergonomics of your bedroom studies have shown best sleep for most is at 65 degrees. People also tend to sleep better if it is in a dry area with a humidifier—no lights, no electronics—unless you are listening to a Calm App. You could also listen to a pre-recorded hypnotic sleep suggestion in your voice. The room needs to be dark. If it is true dark out, but the light is still coming in, you may need more curtain panels or get a better quality of blackout shades.

Ergonomically if you have tried making adjustments and are still not getting proper full sleep, then one question: do you have a pet that sleeps on your bed? The correct ergonomic bedroom would also be one without pets. Are you allergic to them but do not want to admit it? I get it. Getting an air purifier may help. Make sure you can run the air purifier without a light on it disturbing your sleep. Suppose your pet wants to get your attention to get you to pet them consistently. I know it is hard, but slowly, you can transition your pet from sleeping on your bed to sleeping in their bed to sleeping outside your bedroom. It is no easy task when you see your pet's adorable eyes or hear their scratch at the door telling you to let them in. Good luck with this suggestion. It may take a while for this to sink in; patience is key. If you buckle into your pets, you start the process all over again. Pray for willpower.

Studies have shown that being rocked back and forth helps one obtain better sleep. You can visit rockingbed.com. It is an expense, but if you like to enhance your deep sleep even more for restoration and have the spending cash to do so, you could consider it as an option. Studies have shown sleeping in a hammock that also rocks back and forth has its pluses as it helps you breathe better. I have not tried this as I am so enjoying the comfort of the mattress. With a hammock, I'd be afraid of tipping over.

If people ask me the best position to sleep, I would say on your back or left side. On your left side because it may help with digestion. People who are stomach sleepers or side sleepers may have a difficult time changing into this position. An inside hammock could help one transition. The rocking of a hammock may also help one fall asleep quickly.

CHAPTER 6

Ergonomics and Exercise, Your Exercises

With exercises, there are several different types to consider here to help you get sensational sleep. There are postural correcting, meditative breathing, cardiovascular and weight-bearing exercises. Each is helpful in its own way in promoting sensational sleep.

In my office, we use Web-Based Exercises from WebExercises.com to help correct the lopsided weak muscles and recommend myofascial and foam rolling techniques to help relax over worked muscles. The Web-based exercises can work in conjunction with the posture photos to give specific recommendations to help facilitate great posture and reduce pain and ultimately help you even breathe better so you can sleep better. Using a Web Exercises program can tailor what you need to transition you to better outcomes to improved posture.

Some of my posture correcting exercise favorites are:

Head Retraction:

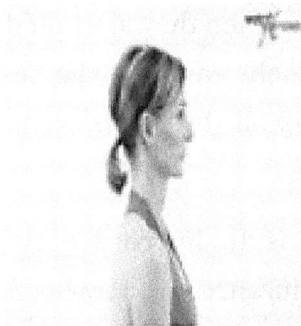

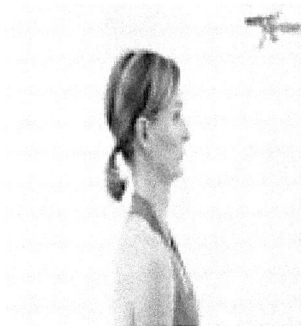

Body Part Neck Muscle(s) Splenius, Semispinalis Capitis, Semispinalis Cervicis, Longissimus Capitis, Longissimus Cervicis, Longus Capitis, and Longus Colli.

Draw head directly backward. Maintain level head position. Hold for two seconds. Return to starting position and repeat for prescribed repetitions and sets. I recommend starting with one set of 10 and work up to three sets of 10. It does not seem like this would be an issue, but I have noticed many people get sore when they start off doing the three sets of 10. It looks easy, but the next day may be painful if doing all three sets when your body is not used to it.

This exercise is to increase neck strength and muscular endurance. You will find improved stability, functional strength, and injury prevention.

Levator Scapula Stretch:

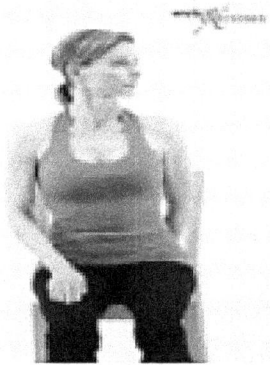

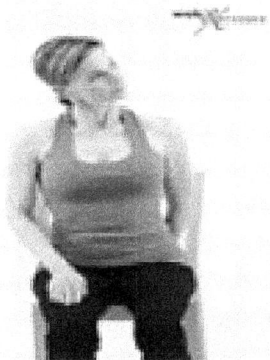

Purpose: correct neck imbalances and restore function. Benefits: increases flexibility, improves joint range of motion, and improves circulation.

Begin seated in chair. Maintain proper sitting posture on sit-bones with shoulders back. Place one hand on your thigh and the other behind your back.

Rotate your head towards the side of your body with the hand behind your back. Then lean head away and down attempting to lower opposite ear to back of hand on thigh providing a stretch to your Levator Scapula, Scalenes, and Trapezius. Hold for 20–30 seconds. Repeat for prescribed repetitions and sets—alternate sides as directed.

This exercise helps correct neck imbalances and restores function. You will find an increase in flexibility, improved joint range of motion, and improved circulation.

Wall Angels:

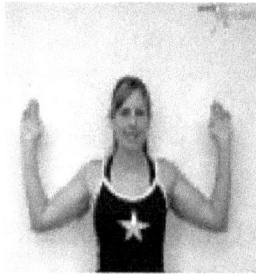

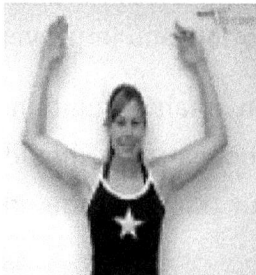

Body Part Mid Back Muscle(s) Deltoid—anterior, Deltoid—lateral, Pec Major—Clavicular head, Supraspinatus, Rhomboid Minor, Upper Back.

Begin standing with shoulder blades flat against the wall. Place arms against the wall with elbows below shoulder level, bent to 90º with palms facing forward.

While attempting to maintain forearm contact with the wall, slide arms upward, squeezing shoulder blades together. Once the forearm can longer maintain contact with the wall, slowly return to the start position. Repeat prescribed repetitions and sets.

This exercise helps to increase mid-back strength and muscular endurance. One will find improved stability, functional strength, and injury prevention.

Bilateral External Rotation with Scapular Retraction:

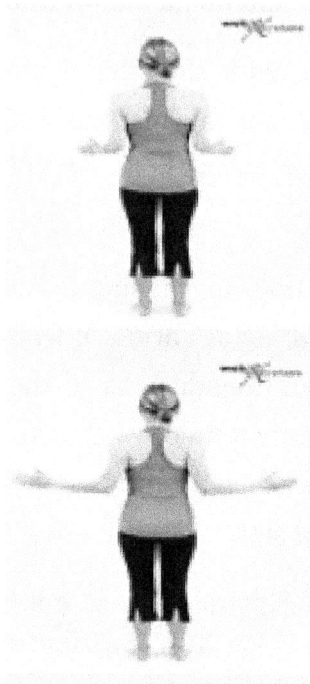

Body Part Mid Back Muscle(s) Teres Major, Teres Minor, Shoulders, Upper Arms, Trapezius middle, Trapezius lower, Rhomboids Major, Rhomboids Minor.

You will find an improvement in stability, functional strength, and injury prevention.

Begin standing in good posture. Shoulders should be back and head up. Bend elbows to 90 degrees and keep elbows near sides.

Keeping great posture, draw shoulders back, squeezing shoulder blades together. Do not allow shoulders to raise upward. Hold for 10 seconds. Repeat for prescribed sets and repetitions.

This exercise helps to increase strength and muscular endurance.

Chest Stretch:

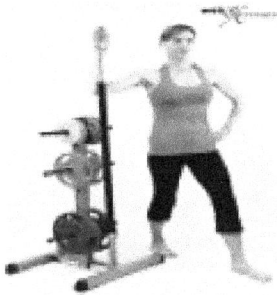

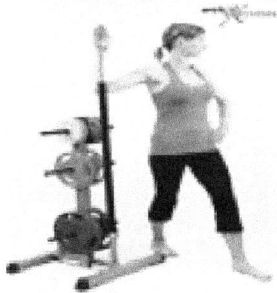

Place forearm on wall next to doorway with elbow bent at 90°. Your elbow should be slightly below shoulder level.

While maintaining forearm contact, rotate your body away until you feel a gentle stretch in the chest and shoulder. Hold for 30 seconds.

The stretch will help to correct muscular imbalances and restore range of motion. You will find an increase in flexibility, and improved mobility and joint function.

Mid Back Myofascial Release:

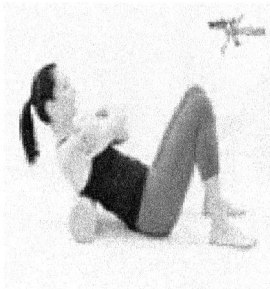

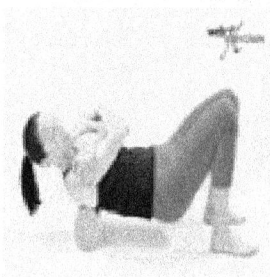

Body Part Mid Back Muscle(s) Trapezius lower, Trapezius middle, Rhomboids Major, Upper Back.

Equipment needed is a foam roller.

Begin with the foam roll in the middle of the back. Cross the arms opening the shoulder blade region, and lift your hips off the floor.

Slowly work the upper back, rolling up and down as tolerated, for a minute or so. If you find a painful area, stop moving and REST on the spot for 10 seconds if you can accept.

The soft tissue work provides deep tissue soft tissue work to correct muscular imbalances. One will find improvements in flexibility, decreased muscle tension, and pain relief.

Breathing Exercises:

Better posture allows better room for breathing, increased motion range, less pain, and increased ability to relax.

We also need to talk about breathing exercises. It should come naturally to breathe correctly. However, suppose you suffer from forward head posture for years and observe yourself. In that case, you may notice when you breathe, your chest is expanding, not your abdominal region like it typically should be doing. A simple test is to put your hand on your chest and the other on top of your navel. You should notice that the abdominal area expands as you breathe in and gets smaller as you exhale. If you see and feel that your chest is rising and falling more than your abdomen, you are shallow breathing, causing your body to work harder to get enough oxygen. If you awaken with a parched mouth, you may also be breathing through your mouth, not your nose. Using the lower part of your lungs by engaging your diaphragm will help you breathe deeply more efficiently and through your nose. Some people feel that their nose is constantly congested, at least in one nostril, if not both. The breathing exercise we will mention over time will help you breathe through your nose and use your lower part of your lungs. Using the lower part of your lungs will help your immune system too clear out debris. If you are stressed and congested, you may notice you are primarily breathing through your mouth. Breathing through your nose allows you to release more nitric oxide, which helps with controling our blood oxygen levels. Air taken in by mouth breathing does not effectively produce nitric oxide. Breathing through your mouth all the time is problematic for sleeping. You will find that the fight or flight response can trigger repetitive mouth breathing. The brain will have the adrenal glands to secrete more adrenalin which causes us to awaken during the night. Other things we could do, but people do not do often enough—saline nasal flush and using a humidifier.

If you are breathing more through the chest, let's look at what we can do to improve our breathing using abdominal muscles and diaphragm. Place one hand on your navel and the other on your chest. Breathe in through the nose for a count of 4. Let your abdominal area expand and hold for 7 and then exhale through your mouth for 8. As you are exhaling, you should notice the abdominal area getting smaller. You can tighten your abdominal muscles to see the effect. There is another breathwork called the Box Breath. You breathe in for 4, hold for 4, exhale for 4 and then pause for 4. The exercise I like is to breath in for 4 and release for 6. This practice sets one up for 6 breaths per minute which studies show this to be optimal to help increase your heart rate variability. Breathing exercises will help strengthen your use of the diaphragm. With a more muscular and functional diaphragm, you will be able to get rid of debris and stale air from the depth of your lungs. Start with doing a set of three for the above breathing exercises and see which one is your favorite.

Yoga. I love yoga because it includes meditative, breathwork, and postural position exercises and stretching and holding yoga. It helps with mindfulness and focusing. There are numerous types of yoga practices in which you can find one that works for you.

Stress becomes more manageable with regular yoga practice. Many studies demonstrate that yoga can improve sleep quality for various populations, particularly for children, pregnant women, women during menopause, and the elderly. Yoga, along with breathing exercises and meditation, has mindfulness as part of the practice. Mindfulness can increase melatonin. Studies have shown that restless leg syndrome reduces with just eight weeks of yoga classes. I remember thinking yoga was to be stretching and relaxing. I went to a power yoga class a few weeks after having my first baby. I did not know it was a moderate to advance exercise. I realized rather quickly how exhausted my body was and that it needed to find a class more suitable for the period that I was in, recovering from having a baby. Read about each type and find the one that will fit you for your level. There are times when we need to start with something simple and work up to something more extensive or a combination of both. Cardiovascular exercises that may include some forms of yoga might be best to do at the beginning of your day or late morning instead of right before bed.

Some of you might be thinking, I have too much arthritis to do any form of exercise. Take note, the less you move, the stiffer you will become. The activities I suggest are swimming and yoga. Swimming—everyone feels better with less pressure on your joints. You can take each joint and typically have a full range of motion in the water than when not in the water. Keeping your range of motion is vital in keeping your ability to move. Don't know how to swim? Take a water aerobics class. Too painful to be on your feet even in the water? Move yourself to the deep end, and do the course by wearing a belt that keeps you afloat. Your range of motion improves, and your pain will lessen. Doing exercises increases your endorphins and you will feel better. The point is to push yourself bit by bit and you will be doing something productive for yourself.

In the past, I would sign myself up for an event such as doing an Alcatraz swim, triathlon event, or a marathon to keep me focused and accountable. At times I would set my mind up to have a specific time for getting Boston Marathon time. However, it does not need to be this grand. It could be a 5 K event, or I will walk around this block in 15 minutes instead of 30 minutes. Find out what works for you. For myself at the time of writing this book I have been walking and hiking in the trails more than running. I am still exercising. At this time, I find the need not to push so hard in this arena. However, I am also getting the itch for an event to occur so I can start training. I feel great when I am training for an event. It is something to look forward to seeing how I come up to the challenge. Keep yourself engaged in some form of physical activity.

I do think mixing it up a bit is fantastic. I have not done so yet, but I like the idea of a Spartan race as it has running and obstacle courses to challenge your strength. I signed up for one in June of 2020 but canceled due to COVID. Bad weather where you live? You could consider purchasing a stationary bike, treadmill, exercise group on demand, or finding your favorite free YouTube videos and get moving. If you start going to bed on time and falling asleep on time, you might be getting up with enough time in the morning to do 20–30 minutes. Something is better than nothing.

What else helps someone with breathing is swimming. With swimming, inhale hold, slowly exhale breathing out hold, and take another breath. That is if you swim correctly. Some people take a breath and hold and are never blow bubbles to exhale the air. You need to exhale the air! Any cardiovascular exercise is going to help tremendously with your deep breathing. Running and biking earlier in the day is an excellent way to get sun and fresh air into your system. However, one that is great to do at night that you can do in your bedroom is having great sex. Besides sleep, the bedroom is for sex. It is the one activity other than sleep that should be allowed in the bedroom. The bedroom is your sanctuary for these two activities.

While orgasms with a partner appear to have the most benefit in terms of sleep outcomes, orgasms achieved through self-stimulation can also aid sleep quality and latency. Sex and Sleep: Perceptions of Sex as a Sleep Promoting Behavior in the General Adult: having sex increases hormones that help promote relaxation; it is a stress reducer and reduces pain—all things that can help you sleep better.

Some people avoid sex because it causes them too much pain, especially if one has spinal cord injury or arthritis. There are positions that you need to discover that will lessen pain and increase your pleasure. It is vital to keep communicating and continue to find positions that work for both of you.

Running, biking, swimming—especially outside in nature trails and open water—is very meditative.

It opens you to see there is more to just the day in day out grind of work. There is an entire another world of adventure of being in nature and discovering a new trail, learning the talent of swimming against a current, finding out ways to improve on your skill of riding your bike downhill and seeing a family of coyotes or listening to the birds or perhaps swimming next to a seal. It is exciting to take your mind off the daily routine and be with nature. It truly helps you to be present when you run in the path of a herd of cows. Being alert as you are running on a new path for different obstacles like a root or rock or mud in the way or riding your bike on a sleek road or swimming, and the current picks up. Doing exercise in nature helps you to stay focused and on top of your game. Taking your mind completely off of everything else and focusing it on something else, like surviving your run without falling, is meditative. It gives you a break. It helps you to realize there is much more than just 9–5 work, etc. Swimming in the cold refreshing water stimulates your Parasympathetic nervous system that helps promote healing and calmness. Spending time outdoors relates to sleeping better, having less pain and more range of motion, and better mood. Being in nature can improve mood, respiratory and cardiovascular diseases, and reduce high blood pressure—all of which help enhance your sleep ability. Being in nature, walking barefoot when you can, or swimming in the open waters helps ground you. Grounding yourself has been shown to help with falling asleep, reducing pain, increasing daytime energy, and lowering cortisol.

Our disconnection from the Earth has helped lead to inflammatory-related chronic diseases. Our bodies that naturally help with our autoimmune response improves with recharging by conductive contact with the Earth.

The number one reason you should exercise in the morning and outside is to set your circadian rhythm optimally. Fresh air and light, along with exercise, are excellent. It helps to promote melatonin naturally. If you exercise in the morning when cortisol levels are higher before you have breakfast, you will burn more fat. It may seem you are so hungry. Try having a glass of water with some lemon, grated ginger, along with a touch of cayenne pepper and filter. This drink helps with inflammation, metabolism, and with you feeling hungry. Great for the morning. If you make a habit and get past this hurdle, your cravings will go down, including your waistline. If you shed the extra weight and don't put on the pounds, it encourages better breathing, better blood pressure, and better sleep.

CHAPTER 7

What Supplements and Nutrition Should I Consider to Help with Sleep?

What supplements and nutrition should I consider to help with sleep? What over-the-counter medications should I avoid? Somebody can write an entire book on this topic. Here I will list some main points in no particular order. As with all supplements, look at a resource such as https://reference.medscape.com/ drug-interactionchecker to confirm no known complications with other supplements or medications you might be taking. If liver problems, pregnant or breastfeeding, seek medical advice. It is equally important to mention that too much of certain nutrients may not be a good thing either. Having a nutritionist help guide you is a great way to help keep you on the right track.

Before we talk about what you could add to, let's first talk about **what you can leave behind**. The first item you know what it is, caffeine.

1. Caffeine

Limit your CAFFEINE to 0 or none 6 hours before bed. Caffeine blocks adenosine receptors. Adenosine is a sleep-promoting chemical that naturally increases the longer we are awake. But if too much caffeine, your build-up of Adenosine reduces, making it longer than usual to fall asleep. Caffeine has a half-life of 6 hours, meaning you digest half of it after 6 hours of what you consumed. If you are seriously having issues with sleep, the caffeine has to go. It is not easy. I suggest slowly cutting back. For instance, if you make your brew, make it 4:1 caffeine to decaffeinate, then to 3:1 ratio, then to half and half caffeine to decaf, and then to 1:4 ratio to finally just one cup of decaf. If you insist on having your cup of joe or other caffeine beverage, you should have the last cup by 6 hours before you're attempting to sleep.

2. Sugar

An excess of sugar creates havoc on our sleep and ultimately our immune system. Sugar consumption depletes magnesium absorption, which you need for optimal sleep.

3. Alcohol

Alcohol may help you fall asleep, but sleep is often disturbed by waking up in the middle of the night to use the restroom and getting a headache— making it hard to fall back to sleep or get deep sleep.

4. Smoking

Are you a smoker? One more reason to quit smoking. It is a stimulant and can make it difficult for you to sleep. You may get light sleep, but the restorative sleep lacks. Stop smoking, and you may find it much easier to get your shut-eye. Smokers also tend to be persistent coffee drinkers. Some people feel smoking is a tension reducer, but studies show it increases anxiety. Smokers also tend to have high blood pressure, tend to snore, and develop sleep apnea. All are making it challenging to get quality sleep. Smoking also affects your musculoskeletal health by increasing inflammation in the body and becoming less tolerable to pain, requiring more medications and more difficulty getting in a comfortable position to fall asleep and stay asleep. The chemicals in a cigarette cause a decrease in oxygen delivery to tissues making a recovery from an injury take longer and more problematic. Are you having difficulty with stopping? Hypnosis helps many people. It might be something you could consider not just with sleep but cutting out habits that lead to poor sleep like smoking.

5. Benadryl

Sleep aids like Benadryl may be beneficial to those with allergies. It can be a temporary solution to help one fall asleep. Still, ultimately, like alcohol, it does not promote the deep restorative sleep you need, and people develop a resistance to using it. If you read some chats online about people having difficulty sleeping, they talk about using several doses nightly to get some shut-eye. You are not having difficulty sleeping because you did not take enough Benadryl. You can only shove so much under the rug before all the mess is exposed. It is crucial to address why you are unable to sleep and correct.

Cutting out caffeine is a great start and helps reduce using sleep aids such as Benadryl to no longer use it. Reducing any of the item can help improve your sleep.

Let's talk about your TIME OF DINNER. It should be 3–4 hours or more before you go to sleep. Consumption of food releases insulin, which signals to be awake in the brain. If you are lying down too soon before your food digests, it can lead to heartburn and make it more difficult to sleep because your body can't relax and sleep when it has another job that takes priority; digestion.

Items to help calm one down—Ashwagandha, tryptophan, chamomile, Valerian Root, magnesium, and lavender. You will need to discover what works for you. Some people are overwhelmed with trying all of these things or taking a whole bunch of stuff. You could try one for 5 days and see how it affects you. If you do not like it, stop and try the next item on the list. For further information on different herbs, I recommend Encyclopedia of Herbal Medicine: 550 Herbs and

Remedies for Common Ailments and Herbal Medicine Insomnia and The 10 Best Solutions to Solve Insomnia Naturally by DB Publishing.

Here are some of the many choices to think about:

Taking OMEGA 3 for inflammation when you have your meal 4–8 hours before you sleep. Taking Omega 3, should be taken with some fat, like an avocado, to help with absorption. You can test your vitamin levels and your omega 3 levels with a blood test to see if you are deficient or borderline.

If you have restless legs and it wakes you up, then check your IRON levels. There has been a link to iron deficiency and restless leg syndrome.

B VITAMINS help with falling asleep and staying asleep.

Increase VITAMIN D: I think is best by increasing your intake of sun with an outdoor activity. Otherwise, look at it in the foods you eat. More sleep, more Melatonin, more Vitamin D and one gets more sensational sleep.

CALCIUM and POTASSIUM if deficient, can result in sleep issues

ZINC, many have a deficiency. Zinc is a sleep modulator. One way to tell if you have enough of it is to take a small sip of it. If it tastes like nothing, you don't have enough of it. Consider adding zinc.

IODINE: if you are wired and tired, it might be your thyroid. You may have hypothyroid, or you may not be getting enough iodine. There is an inexpensive way to check if you have enough of this as well. Purchase an iodine tincture. Put the solution on a cotton ball and make a 3-inch by 3-inch patch on your arm. A sign that you have iodine deficiency is if the patch fades sooner than 24 hours.

CBD helps decrease cortisol levels, 300–600 mg of CBD oil may help act as a sedative.

MAGNESIUM MANGANESE CITRATE is easily absorbed and helps your muscles relax, and it also helps with melatonin production.

MELATONIN helps you fall asleep faster. You should be able to produce enough if you get exposed to light during the day. Jet lag—using Melatonin can help you get to your new schedule. As we age our ability to produce Melatonin declines. If you want to continue to get great sleep, sleep helps to detoxify your brain, then taking it can help you in many ways. Some may be wary of taking it because they think the body will produce less on its own if taking a supplement. However, studies have shown taking in doses of 10 mg does not interfere with your body's production.

CHAMOMILE has the antioxidant apigenin that binds to specific receptors in your brain that help you sleep.

VALERIAN ROOT: Valerian helps reduce the breakdown of GABA, so one tends to stay calm. It helps promote Serotonin, so one feels peaceful and very relaxed. 300–600 mg 1–2 hours before sleeping has improved the quality of sleep.

ASHWAGANDHA is an adaptogen. It is one of the favorites as it helps to reduce anxiety by lowering your sensitivity to stress and therefore allowing you to relax.

LAVENDER: these compounds inhibit several neurotransmitters and have a sedative and pain-relieving effect, lowers the heart rate and reduces anxiety.

BIOIDENTICAL HORMONES may help the woman during menopausal time. The reduction in Estrogen and Progesterone can promote insomnia. By getting these items in balance can help one sleep better. Some may say we are supposed to get older. Others can also argue nature has not caught up to the fact we are living longer. Living longer, you will age better with great sleep. A naturopathic doctor can do a urine sample Dutch test and help you get your system to balance. It is up to you to make the final decision. Low Testosterone in men may contribute to insomnia as well. Being under care with a trained professional can help you get the correct dosage that is right for you.

TRYPTOPHAN is an amino acid that can converts into Serotonin and Melatonin, helping with mood and sleep.

SAFFRON study showed no reported adverse effects of taking 14 mg twice a day for 28 days with self-reported sleep quality improvement.

PREBIOTICS AND PROBIOTICS/LEAKY GUT AND VAGUS NERVE AND INSOMNIA Intestinal metabolism is connected to brain function by the circulatory system and Vagus nerve—a network called the brain-gut axis. The Vagus nerve leaves the medulla oblongata extended to the neck, chest, abdomen, and the colon. The Vagus nerve consists mainly of afferent nerves relaying sensory information from the organs to the central nervous system. Research shows that the gut microbiome affects our brain function and circadian rhythm. If you rid your gut of the toxins, eat clean, eat foods with probiotics and prebiotics, you may help yourself fall asleep faster and maybe stay asleep longer.

CBD, cannabis helps with many different items such as sleep and anxiety and help reduce inflammation, thus less pain and easier to fall asleep. Some companies make it in different forms like gummies that you can even have Melatonin added to it. Some you sample under your tongue, and when it tastes sweet as honey, this is the proper dosage for you. Also, CBD comes in cream form to help with pain in the neck and body complaints, and it sells quickly off my shelf. It helps right at the area. It is nice to use in conjunction with soft tissue work. It smells terrific too!

The one that I have been taking is Melatonin. I have to be honest, at first, I was hesitant because the theory is the more you take something your body makes, the less your body will produce that ingredient. The truth is, as we get older, we have a reduction in Melatonin production. You can do things to help promote your natural ability. For those over the age of 50 or for jet lag, Melatonin studies demonstrated that taking .5mg to 5mg of Melatonin a night 2 hours before sleep DOES NOT reduce your ability to produce Melatonin.

Melatonin naturally will increase by getting off of the electronics and going camping. If that is not an option, you could also force yourself to rise when the sun rises and also see the sunset. Reducing the caffeine intake will help with Melatonin production as well.

Eating a well-balanced diet is helpful. Keeping your weight under control is crucial to you being able to breathe easier while you sleep and allow you a deeper sleep. Sleep apnea occurs mainly with one being overweight.

I also believe that people are not getting enough water. You should consume half your body weight in ounces daily, especially if you are an athlete; you may need more. Drinking enough water helps you to flush out toxins and helps your body transport nutrients.

DNA-based nutrition is something you may want to consider. There is DNA-based nutrition where they take a sample of your saliva, give you a report and then design nutritional supplements for you. DNA-based nutrition can be beneficial since it gives you valuable items to help you combat diseases and inflammation that you are prone to inherit. There are more and more advances coming along our way with nutrition. Even with testing to see if you are prone to anxiety and then developing nutrition to help you feel better. It is customized for you, so the guesswork is out of the picture.

One can help balance their hormones with diet and exercise. However, if you are middle-aged and going through having difficulty sleeping, then Bioidentical Hormones might be a solution for you. Bioidentical hormones you can use to get you back to feeling yourself. I do believe that mother nature has not caught up with the fact that we are, for the most part, living longer. Taking bioidentical hormones and even Melatonin is one way to help you look and feel great. If you want to live longer, feeling younger and looking longer, and have your organs function well, it may be something to investigate for yourself. I know I used to be on the fence on this.

I thought we are supposed to go through change and getting older is part of life. For some, transition is easy. For others, more complicated, perhaps your nutrition and exercise and sleeping habits you have are good. For others, if you have insomnia during this time, it is one item to consider. Studies show benefits to taking bioidentical hormones are numerous from helping you with sleep, reduce anxiety and how your brain and your other organs function. I have concluded I am planning on living a long time feeling my best and have great restorative sleep to be productive for as long as possible. The book, The Sexy Years: Discover the Hormone Connection: The Secret to Fabulous Sex, Great Health, and Vitality, for

Women and Men by Suzanne Somers is a great read and opened my eyes to a different perspective. Each individual will need to make this decision if it is suitable for them or not. The first thing I noticed taking progesterone was better sleep. Also, skin texture much smoother. Look for a doctor specializing in bioidentical hormones. Naturopathic doctors can also prescribe these hormones. Many naturopathic doctors' nutrition is their top expertise. There are always risks, and that is something you will need to assess.

Some people have what they call a leaky gut. Some of the large intestine bacteria have gone up into the small intestine, invading with a different type of bacteria that is not normally found in the small intestine, becoming problematic. It turns out that the bacteria reinforce your system via sending signals to your brain via the Vagus nerve to eat more of certain types of food such as gluten and sugar. I am not kidding you when these "harmful "bacteria hijack your system and give messages via the Vagus nerve and relates to your hypothalamus and limbic system providing information on what one needs to produce and what not to produce. If enough harmful bacteria develop, they send the wrong information up, basically telling your system you are craving sugary and gluten types of food. Getting rid of this issue is no easy task.

You need to stop eating sugar, refined foods, etc.— easier said than done. It may help you fall asleep faster like alcohol, but the restorative sleep quality significantly lessens, and one may end up craving more sugar. An increase in sugar can increase inflammation, in turn causing havoc on your sleep cycle.

What TO eat and drink:

Drink half your weight in oz. of WATER every day. Consume primarily vegetables, fruit, quality meat, and quality fats such as seeds, nuts, avocado, coconut oil, and olive oil. The Mediterranean Diet is one to consider. If you are going to eat animal protein, it's best if you can get organic humanely raised and grass-fed grass-finished—these are higher in quality of containing Omega 3s plus a list of several other bonuses.

L-Glutamine, 1,500 mg of l-glutamine per serving, and Licorice Root, 150 to 400 mg dosage, helps control Helicobacter pylori. These harmful bacteria can enter your body through your digestive tract, causing inflammation and ultimately ulcers. Acacia fiber gum, a soluble fiber, helps heal your intestine wall. Also, taking prebiotics and probiotics, which I will explain in a moment, is helpful. DNA-based nutrition will likely already have this as a natural part of its ingredients.

If you suspect you have SIBO, small intestinal bacterial overgrowth, seeking out an honest naturopathic doctor or nutritionist would be a wise decision. The typical test done in the medical doctor's office won't pick it up. Breath testing will determine if you have harmful bacteria in your small intestine. It is non-intrusive and used to help determine if you have SIBO. The test works by testing for hydrogen or methane in the breath at specific times after a person drinks a sugary solution. More sugar, more gluten equals less sleep. Our gut microbiome also has a say in the working of your body and brain through triggering the release of hormones or producing them.

The bacteria can communicate with your nervous system, and certain types affect your production of serotonin. By reducing your serotonin levels, the gut bacteria can interfere with your sleep. Your brain and your gut can enter a vicious circle when it comes to sleep, as poor sleep can hurt your gut health. When your serotonin levels reduce without a correct microbiome, it results in less sleep. An incorrect microbiome relates to a more bulging stomach that can put pressure on your diaphragm, making it more difficult to breathe, primarily when you lie down to sleep. Therefore, more likely mouth breathing, which ultimately ends with less deep restorative sleep. Studies on mice found that mice with microbes from the Clostridiaceae and Peptostreptococcaceae families help with fat absorption allowing one to gain weight. The abundance of other bacteria such as Bifidobacteriacaea and Bacteriodacaea are associated with the decreased ability to absorb fat resulting in a much leaner body. When germ-free mice are introduced to microbes that contribute to fat digestion, they quickly gained weight.

Prebiotics such as green tea and high-quality dark chocolate, asparagus, beans, and plums help with your sleep quality.

Probiotics are healthy bacteria and can be found in live kimchi and sauerkraut or taken in powder form to promote beneficial bacteria. Taking both prebiotics and probiotics helps reduce inflammation and improve your metabolism.

I need to mention that most do not take enough of the Omega-3 oils. Having more of them helps reduce inflammation and taking this with Boswellia and Turmeric is a great combination to help reduce the inflammation in the body and ultimately with pain. With less pain you will find it easier to find a comfortable position to sleep in and hence fall asleep faster and stay asleep.

CHAPTER 8

What Do You Mean by Take Out?

What do you mean by take out? Want to make your sleep sensational? Then take a clear look and inventory of what is going on in your life and start making some changes. Some may want one-to-one coaching. I admit it would be easier to have one right there going through everything. That is something that sleep coaches do offer privately, or sometimes it is better in a group setting. However, I challenge you to do this first on your own. See how far you can clean this up. I know you can do this. That is, if your sleep is bad enough, do it. Some people keep going down a rabbit hole so far down that it is difficult to get out. Perhaps you are taking tons of Benadryl to give you some shut-eye after all the caffeine you had during the day. Your life can be a lot different; you need to choose it. It is like drug addicts; they go so far until they wake up and clean up or don't wake up.

First, let's summarize the bedroom. Is your room super busy and colorful with a lot going on, or is it calm and soothing? Do you still have the TV in your room? Take it out! What about the computer, phone, iPad, etc.? I strongly encourage you to get these out of your space. If you cannot because you are in a dorm, turn off the Wi-Fi, Bluetooth, and cellular an hour before you sleep. If you can see your electronics lying in your room, you might want to consider putting them behind a wall or divider. So one side is for working or homework and the other side for sleeping. If you share a room, you might need to get eyeshades, and if there is someone who snores, you might have to get earplugs. Encourage them, however, to seek out a sleep study from their doctor.

Is there any light in your room when you close the blinds or curtains? Not all black out shades are created equally. There should be no light popping through. Maybe you need to get true black out shades or purchase more panels so that outside light stops coming into the bedroom. Are you stuffy at night and find it hard to breathe through your nose? Is it your carpet? Is it full of dust? When was the last time you had it steam cleaned? Best if you can get rid of carpet altogether, but if not, get it cleaned, invest in the iRobot Roomba, and have it clean under your bed. What type of mattress covering, and pillowcases are you using? Do they keep you protected from bed bugs? How often are you washing your sheets that you lay your head on? Weekly, I hope. Are you sleeping with your pets? Do you notice that they are keeping you up? It might be best to snuggle with them on the couch and to train them now so you can sleep better. Difficult to do?

Invest in the pet trainer. Have you done this, and you still seem to have allergies when you lay down at night? Invest in the expensive air filter for allergies. You know the one, Filtrete for allergy sufferers. Invest in this stuff; it is for your well-being. Are you finding it difficult to get comfortable because your bed sinks in and is so old? Invest in a new one like 360 air number bed or try a hybrid one. At least get a mattress topper to see if that helps if too firm or put extra support under the mattress if too soft. Waking up with neck pain? Get rid of your pillow, and at least keep searching for the pillow that works for you. I currently like the core pillow. You can take out the material to get it to make sure it is accurate for your neck's restore curvature. The point is to discover what works for you. If your bed has been up against the same wall and you have not been getting good sleep, change it around and place it in the new position. State throughout the week with this position of my bed, I get sensational sleep. The thoughts you state in your head are potent. Believe it to be accurate and see what happens. What else happens at night? When you lay down, and all of these thoughts go on in your head, what do you do? Take yourself out of the room, for Pete's sake. Get your sensational sleep journal and write it in there and start doing that nightly. At the end of your entry, write, may I dream of something sweet that guides me to observe this situation with possible solutions. Then in the morning, see if you remember any dream. Please write it down, look it up in dream interpreter, and see if your dream provides some clarity for you. If anything, you will have a new hobby.

Are you waking up hot as ever, and you know it is not your hormones? Then take out the heat! Keep your bedroom at 65 degrees and find out what temperature works best for you by journaling nights of great sleep and what was the temperature set on. Do you have fake plants in your room? Full of dust? Try investing in some great house plants living that help with sleep. Some help clean the air of toxins such as formaldehyde from carpets. Some plants release oxygen at night. See if having a plant in your room seems to help you rest or keeps you up. If you are not getting sensational sleep, change the environment, and again with this change throughout the day state it in your head, write it down and even state it aloud. The bed in this position helps me sleep easily. These plants in this room clean the air and help me breathe easily through my nose. These changes help promote great sleep. See what happens in a week? Are you sleeping better? By taking care of the plant in your room, you symbolize taking care of yourself.

Now let us take a look at the kitchen. What is in it? Alcohol? If you need help with this item, seek out AA, and a great counselor might be helpful too. Honestly, I have taken inventory that if I have more than one glass of wine, I do not get good sleep, and I wake up with a headache that lasts for a couple of days! You have one drink. It feels so good to decide; well, that was good, maybe another one will even be better. Hey, if you can't say no to only one, it might be better to say none. What else is in the kitchen? Sugar items with corn and modified, processed items—toss them out.

Take out eating 3–4 hours before bed. Have you been trying to sleep after you just ate? Horrible—it creates heartburn. Are you working late? Think about a more substantial lunch and maybe a shake at night.

Take out bright lights 2–3 hours before sleep. Invest in some eyeshades, or it might be easier to set the computer light to dim.

What else can you take out? Let me ask you. Did you check out what your top 3 strengths are at www.viacharacter.com? Are you implementing your strengths in your day-to-day activities? Is it at your work? Is there something you need to switch so you can use your strengths more efficiently?

We are all here for a purpose. I believe with your top 3 strengths you should be finding a way to implement them in your work and hobbies. Is there something you are doing that is keeping you from using your gifts? During the pandemic, many took an inventory of what matters. Many invested in themselves, learning another way to make an additional income. Have you started? Perhaps you are set in your ways at your work, but you do not find it fulfilling. Is there some project you can do that will use your talents? Maybe at a community organization? Or perhaps an event you set up yourself?

On the flip side, maybe you need to take out your bike from the garage and start biking to work or take out the yoga mat and start using it daily to stretch. Maybe you need to take off your shoes and walk barefoot on the ground for 30 minutes, weather permitting, outside to ground yourself. Do you think this is farfetched? It is not. Numerous studies demonstrate how being barefoot on the earth stabilizes your electrical system in your body. Having the connection with the ground with our bare feet helps you balance your electrical activity in you. Grounding yourself helps your immune response. We have gone away from nature. You want sensational sleep, consider grounding. You might even wish to get a mattress that grounds you or get sheets that help ground you.

Highly strung? You might instantly start sleeping a lot better once you unplug. Take yourself off the grid for a weekend. Go camping where there are no electronics. You will find that you are sleeping much earlier.

Simply if you are not sleeping well, take out what is not working for you.

CHAPTER 9

Putting It All Together with R.E.S.T. for Sensational Sleep

Putting it all together with R.E.S.T. for sensational sleep. At the beginning of this book, if you start implementing the R.E.S.T. guideline, you will see an improvement in your sleep, and with continued focus, you will obtain sensational sleep. If you sleep well, you wake up and feel sensational.

Take Caroline, for example, and see if you can relate. Caroline was under a lot of stress. She drank coffee throughout the day and was having difficulty falling asleep. Caroline started taking 1 Benadryl a night which worked but only for 4 hours. Sometimes taking one wasn't enough, so she took 2. Sometimes that would not even work. She was resistant to take any more than that. She went for several days without getting enough sleep. In the morning she was still wired. She quickly gave up caffeine out of necessity. I think she noticed she never even got any headaches that she typically would when cutting out caffeine in the past. As long as she was at work and busy, she's terrific. She started getting worried though not getting enough sleep; eventually, she's going to have to crash. Hopefully, it wouldn't be at the time when she's driving. She even started to panic driving on the way home, going into her place, knowing that she's going to have to try to go to sleep in just a short time. She went to try E.M.D.R. and started recommended sleep routine and started documenting her sleep and daily habits and thoughts. Within a week, she was doing much better and was able to stop taking the Benadryl. She then started to implement her strengths she listed from her quiz in her work and started looking for other ways to implement her strengths daily. She looked at her workstation, moved items around there and in her bedroom to help facilitate better ergonomics, so less pain more comfort, including ditching her pillow for a *Core Pillow*. She started regularly going to her chiropractor and massage therapist instead of waiting until she could not take the pain anymore. She noticed she had fewer flare-ups with getting routine checks. She had a posture screen done and could see for herself how forward her neck was from often sitting with her head forward and how her shoulder tilts from leaning out with her right shoulder with the mouse for her computer. She set up her workstation correctly and got specifics exercises to help with her forward head posture. She was getting about 6 to 7 hours of sleep after about three weeks. There was a big improvement from a short time ago where she was getting as little as 4 hours of sleep a night. Since she was starting menopause and wanted to improve her sleep even more, she started taking bioidentical hormones and a low dosage of melatonin. She took a D.N.A. test and got nutrition based on her genetics. She looked at her bedroom setup to figure out why she did not get a good sleep and what she should do to improve the room to help her sleep. She took note that the bed was too close to her window, so she moved it. She put her phone on airplane mode. She continued to monitor her sleep journal and closely looked at it when having difficulty sleeping to pinpoint what kept her up. She made notes as to when she slept well and what was right. She started to remember more and more of her dreams and what they symbolized to her. It became a fun and artistic expression she felt that came from her dreams. Every night, she looked forward to getting sensational sleep and waking up alert and delighted to start the new day. She has learned through her practice to be an observer of her experiences instead of becoming all consumed.

She found a few mantras that she would say throughout the day, and she made a few of her own such as I sleep soundly, easily, and wake refreshed and ready to start the day. Sensational sleep for a stunning day. On days where she had a lot of stress, she would remind herself with mantra "tonight I will discover answers to my questions with my dreams". She made a self hypnosis recording to help her at night relax and talk about how grateful she is to have the strengths she has and the ability to use them throughout the day. She became calm during the day and not angry all the time. Things that typically would upset her she would notice and have the ability to not let them bother her because she ultimately was content. She felt fantastic with sensational sleep. She had less pain and found that she could recover quicker after a workout that generally would have taken her a few days of complaining. People were happy to hang out with her as her sensational happiness rubbed off on them. She also noticed that she could focus and get things accomplished throughout the day instead of being scattered.

If Caroline can do it, why don't you give it a try? You picked up this book because of issues you are having with sleep. You can start the day right by getting your sensational sleep. Start today with R, your Routine that is a Must. Then implement Ergonomics and exercise. Consider, if needed, bioidentical hormones, melatonin, CBD. D.N.A. nutrition—take out what is not helping you with your sleep . . . such as light curtains.

Are you tired of having difficulty sleeping? Are you sick and tired of lying in bed tossing and turning?

Are you starting to get anxious about going to sleep? Do you forget things? Are you gaining weight but not eating any more than usual? Is it difficult for you to recover from working out? Do you feel like you are always in pain? Are you moody? These are signs you are not sleeping well.

If you are having difficulty sleeping, I challenge you to pick an item from the REST guideline and see what happens to you.

R - Routine a M.U.S.T. (Meditative, Under Accountability, Strengths, and Timely)

E - Ergonomics and Exercise

S - Supplements

T - Take Out what is not working

Will you start on your routine tonight? If you are serious about getting sensational sleep, start with your routine.

Have you implemented R.E.S.T. and want to improve your sleep more? In that case, you could seek out a therapist for E.M.D.R., Eye Movement Desensitization Reprocessing, or a Cognitive Behavioral Therapist—both having great results. If you think sleep apnea is a problem, consider consulting with a dentist to see if bite is an issue and a sleep study. If you are still having difficulty falling asleep and staying asleep because of back pain, isn't it time for you to seek your local chiropractor?

I hope you have enjoyed this book and can implement the REST steps for Sensational sleep. For a free sleep journal download, go to www. sensationalsleepbook.com.

Presentations in person and online are available.

For more information, visit sensationalsleepbook.com.

MY SOURCES:

Suni, Eric. 2020. "What Is Circadian Rhythm?" Sleep Foundation. September 25, 2020. https://www.sleepfoundation.org/circadian-rhythm.

Slouched Posture, Sleep Deprivation, and Mood Disorders: Interconnection and Modulation by Theta Brain Waves/Emma A. Barr1*, Erik Peper2, and Ronald J. Swatzyna1 https://www.neuroregulation.org/article/view/19578.

Jacobson, Malia. 2020. "Oh, so THIS Is Why You Can't Sleep on Race Day." Runner's World. May 11, 2020.

https://www.runnersworld.com/training/a20785
975/is-insomnia-while-training-normal/.

Burke, Tina M., Rachel R. Markwald, Andrew W.
McHill, Evan D. Chinoy, Jesse A. Snider, Sara C.
Bessman, Christopher M. Jung, John S. O'Neill, and
Kenneth P. Wright. 2015. "Effects of Caffeine on
the Human Circadian Clock in Vivo and in Vitro."
Science Translational Medicine 7 (305):
305ra146–46.
https://doi.org/10.1126/scitranslmed.aac5125.ht
tps://jcsm.aasm.org/doi/10.5664/jcsm.3170

Drake, Christopher, Timothy Roehrs, John
Shambroom, and Thomas Roth. 2013. "Caffeine
Effects on Sleep Taken 0, 3, or 6 Hours before
Going to Bed." Journal of Clinical Sleep Medicine
09 (11). https://doi.org/10.5664/jcsm.3170.

Beta-amyloid* Shokri-Kojori, E., Wang, G. J., Wiers,
C. E., Demiral, S. B., Guo, M., Kim, S. W., Lindgren, E.,
Ramirez, V., Zehra, A., Freeman, C., Miller, G.,
Manza, P., Srivastava, T., De Santi, S., Tomasi, D.,
Benveniste, H., & Volkow, N. D. (2018). β-Amyloid
accumulation in the human brain after one night of
sleep deprivation. Proceedings of the National
Academy of Sciences of the United States of

America, 115(17), 4483–4488.
https://doi.org/10.1073/pnas.1721694115

Yang, Rui-Hua, San-Jue Hu, Yuan Wang, Wen-Bin
Zhang, Wen-Jing Luo, and Jing-Yuan Chen. 2008.
"Paradoxical Sleep Deprivation Impairs Spatial
Learning and Affects Membrane Excitability and
Mitochondrial Protein in the Hippocampus." Brain
Research 1230 (September): 224–32.
https://doi.org/10.1016/j.brainres.2008.07.033.

Walker, Matthew P. 2018. Why We Sleep:
Unlocking the Power of Sleep and Dreams. New
York, Ny: Scribner, An Imprint Of Simon &
Schuster, Inc.

Neckelmann, Dag, Arnstein Mykletun, and Alv A.
Dahl. 2007. "Chronic Insomnia as a Risk Factor for
Developing Anxiety and Depression." Sleep 30 (7):
873–80. https://doi.org/10.1093/sleep/30.7.873.

Dinges, D. F., F. Pack, K. Williams, K. A. Gillen, J. W.
Powell, G. E. Ott, C. Aptowicz, and A. I. Pack. 1997.
"Cumulative Sleepiness, Mood Disturbance, and
Psychomotor Vigilance Performance Decrements
during a Week of Sleep Restricted to 4-5 Hours per

Night." Sleep 20 (4): 267–77.
https://pubmed.ncbi.nlm.nih.gov/9231952/.

Prather, Aric A., Denise Janicki-Deverts, Martica H.
Hall, and Sheldon Cohen. 2015. "Behaviorally
Assessed Sleep and Susceptibility to the Common
Cold." Sleep 38 (9): 1353–59.
https://doi.org/10.5665/sleep.4968.

Irwin, M, J McClintick, C Costlow, M Fortner, J
White, and J C Gillin. 1996. "Partial Night Sleep
Deprivation Reduces Natural Killer and Cellular
Immune Responses in Humans." The FASEB
Journal 10 (5): 643–53.
https://doi.org/10.1096/fasebj.10.5.8621064.

Schwarz, P., W. Graham, F. Li, M. Locke, and J.
Peever. 2013. "Sleep Deprivation Impairs
Functional Muscle Recovery Following Injury."
Sleep Medicine 14 (December): e262.
https://doi.org/10.1016/j.sleep.2013.11.638.

Ferrie, Jane E., Martin J. Shipley, Francesco P.
Cappuccio, Eric Brunner, Michelle A. Miller, Meena
Kumari, and Michael G. Marmot. 2007. "A
Prospective Study of Change in Sleep Duration:
Associations with Mortality in the Whitehall II

Cohort." Sleep 30 (12): 1659–66.
https://www.ncbi.nlm.nih.gov/pmc/articles/PMC
2276139/.

Norah Simpson, MA, David F. Dinges, PhD, Sleep
and Inflammation, Nutrition Reviews, Volume 65,
Issue suppl_3, December 2007, Pages S244–S252,
https://academic.oup.com/nutritionreviews/artic
le/65/suppl_3/S244/1911960

Hublin, Christer, Markku Partinen, Markku
Koskenvuo, and Jaakko Kaprio. 2007. "Sleep and
Mortality: A Population-Based 22-Year Follow-up
Study." Sleep 30 (10): 1245–53.
https://doi.org/10.1093/sleep/30.10.1245

"Sleep-Tracking Devices: Dos and Don'ts." n.d.
Mayo Clinic. Accessed April 16, 2021.
https://www.mayoclinic.org/healthy-
lifestyle/adult-health/in-depth/sleep-tracking-
devices-dos-donts/art-20481371.

"Do Sleep Trackers Really Work?" n.d.
Www.hopkinsmedicine.org.
https://www.hopkinsmedicine.org/health/wellne
ss-and-prevention/do-sleep-trackers-really-work.

De Zambotti, Massimiliano, Nicola Cellini, Aimee Goldstone, Ian M. Colrain, and Fiona C. Baker.2019 "Wearable Sleep Technology in Clinical and Research Settings." Medicine & Science in Sports & Exercise 51 (7): 1538–57. https://www.ncbi.nlm.nih.gov/pmc/articles/PMC 6579636/

Espie, Colin A., Richard Emsley, Simon D. Kyle, Christopher Gordon, Christopher L. Drake, A. Niroshan Siriwardena, John Cape, et al. 2019. "Effect of Digital Cognitive Behavioral Therapy for Insomnia on Health, Psychological Well-Being, and Sleep-Related Quality of Life: A Randomized Clinical Trial." JAMA Psychiatry 76 (1): 21. https://jamanetwork.com/journals/jamapsychiat ry/fullarticle/2704019

Bayer, Laurence, Irina Constantinescu, Stephen Perrig, Julie Vienne, Pierre-Paul Vidal, Michel Mühlethaler, and Sophie Schwartz. 2011. "Rocking Synchronizes Brain Waves during a Short Nap." Current Biology 21 (12): R461–62. https://www.sciencedirect.com/science/article/p ii/S0960982211005392#app2

"Rocking Bed | Improve Your Sleep Tonight." n.d. Rocking Bed. Accessed April 16, 2021. https://rockingbed.com/.

"Digital Provider Education & Corrective Exercise Platform." n.d. WebExercises. Accessed April 16, 2021. https://www.webexercises.com/.

"Box Breathing: How to Do It, Benefits, and Tips." 2018. Www.medicalnewstoday.com. June 1, 2018. https://www.medicalnewstoday.com/articles/32 1805#the-box-breathing-method.

Lastella, Michele, Catherine O'Mullan, Jessica L. Paterson, and Amy C. Reynolds. 2019. "Sex and Sleep: Perceptions of Sex as a Sleep Promoting Behavior in the General Adult Population." Frontiers in Public Health 7 (March). https://www.frontiersin.org/articles/10.3389/fp ubh.2019.00033/3.

Oschman, James, Gaetan Chevalier, and Richard Brown. 2015. "The Effects of Grounding (Earthing) on Inflammation, the Immune Response, Wound Healing, and Prevention and Treatment of Chronic Inflammatory and Autoimmune Diseases." Journal of Inflammation Research, March, 83.

https://www.ncbi.nlm.nih.gov/pmc/articles/PMC4378297/

Chevallier, Andrew. 2000. Encyclopedia of Herbal Medicine: The Definitive Home Reference Guide to 550 Key Herbs with All Their Uses as Remedies for Common Ailments. London; New York: Dorling Kindersley.

DB Publishing. August 27, 2018. Herbal Medicine Insomnia: The 10 Best Solutions to Solve Insomnia Naturally

Lopresti, Adrian L, Stephen J Smith, Alexandra P Metse, and Peter D Drummond. 2020. "Effects of Saffron on Sleep Quality in Healthy Adults with Self-Reported Poor Sleep: A Randomized, Double-Blind, Placebo-Controlled Trial." Journal of Clinical Sleep Medicine, February. https://pubmed.ncbi.nlm.nih.gov/32056539/

Lars P. H. Andersen, corresponding author Mads U. Werner, Mette M. Rosenkilde, Nathja G. Harpsøe, Hanne Fuglsang, Jacob Rosenberg, and Ismail Gögenur "Pharmacokinetics of oral and intravenous melatonin in healthy volunteers"Journal of BMC Pharmacolgy and

Toxicolgy, February 2016
https//ncbi.nlminih.gov/pmc/articles/PMC47597
23

Easton, John. 2018. "Specific Bacteria in the Small
Intestine Are Crucial for Fat Absorption."
Uchicagomedicine.org. UChicago Medicine. April
10, 2018.
https://www.uchicagomedicine.org/forefront/gas
trointestinal-articles/specific-bacteria-in-the-
small-intestine-are-crucial-for-fat-absorption.

About the Author

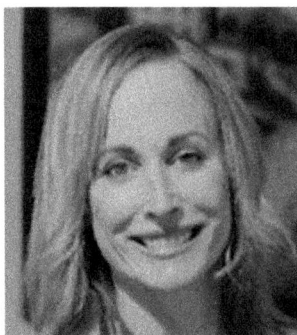

Stacey Duckett is a chiropractor, an applied clinical nutritionist, and a certified hypnotist. She has a certificate for completion on The Science of Well-Being, Series of challenges designed to increase your happiness and build more productive habits from Yale University and Certification in Sleep: Neurobiology, Medicine, and Society, from the University of Michigan, Ann Arbor, Michigan. With her discovery of what works for a night of better sleep, she has written *Sensational Sleep*. As a Doctor of Chiropractic since 1993 and dealing with patients recovering from injuries, she realized that a lot was due to nutrition and exercise and sleep habits. Patients with proper sleep tend to recover quicker from injuries. Ones with chronic pain tend to have improper sleep habits. Stacey noticed training for marathons as she was getting older. She was getting sorer than what would be typical. As one age, especially the female during menopause, she is likely to get less sleep. With less sleep, one tends to have more headaches, more pain, gain weight, mood swings affecting their relationships, and less cognitive ability affecting their work. There is a cascade of reasons why one has issues with sleep, which is imperative to help with the solution. Taking medicine in the short term for specific reasons can be beneficial, but it becomes a crutch with consequences to their overall health in the long term. She found that by improving her sleep habits, nutrition, and ergonomics, she improved both the quality and quantity of sleep. Waking up daily feeling excited about the day with alertness, increasing cognition, improved metabolism, and exercising without the extra pain, she decided on sharing what helps sensational sleep with others to help improve their quality of life in so many ways.

Would you like Stacey Duckett to be a guest speaker at your next event?

Visit **SensationalSleepBook.com**

FREE Sleep Assessment!

www.SensationalSleepBook.com

Would you like to get better sleep?

- Free Sleep Assessment
- Free Sleep Journal pdf
- Sign Up for FREE Email updates

Stacey Duckett, DC, ACN, CH is available to speak at your business or conference event.

Visit www.Sensational SleepBook.com

www.ingramcontent.com/pod-product-compliance
Lightning Source LLC
Chambersburg PA
CBHW060020050426
42448CB00012B/2829